FIBROID FREEDOM

Empowering Women's Wellness through Natural Approach and Holistic Healing.

By

Zoe Peterson

About The Author

Zoe Peterson is the author of "fibroid freedom: Empowering Women's Wellness through Natural Approach and Holistic Healing." She's a renowned health advocate and Researcher, known for her expertise in women's reproductive health. Through her book, she empowers women with valuable insights to combat fibroids, offering hope and practical solutions.

Table of Contents

PREFACE

Welcome to the transformative journey within the pages of "Fibroid Freedom: Empowering Women's Wellness through Natural Approach and Holistic Healing." This book is an empowering guide for those facing the challenges of fibroids. Witting these chapters, you will find not only knowledge but also the keys to taking control of your health. We explore that causes, symptoms, and treatment of fibroids, embracing a holistic approach that recognizes the profound connection between mind and body. As you read on, May you uncover the strength within you to make informed choices and embark on a path towards wellness, freedom and empowerment in your health journey.

INTRODUCTION

Welcome to "Fibroid Freedom: Empowering Women's wellness through Natural Approach and Holistic Healing." In the pages of this book, we embark on a journey to unravel the mysteries surrounding fibroids and explore the pathways to holistic healing and empowerment.

Fibroids, though common, often hide in the shadows of women's health conversations. These benign growths can impact our lives in ways that extend far beyond their physical presence. In this introduction, we'll delve into the world of fibroids, understanding their origins, the challenges they pose, and the inspiration that drives us to seek a comprehensive solution.

We'll peer into the conventional medical perspectives on fibroids, gaining insights into the diagnostic processes and treatment options available. As we navigate these insights, we'll also shine a light on the limitations and potential side effects of traditional approaches, laying the foundation for the exploration of alternative paths.

Holistic healing takes center stage as we examine the intricate interplay between our bodies, minds, and lifestyles. From nutrition's role in managing fibroids to the connection between stress and hormone balance, we'll uncover the potential of natural remedies and lifestyle adjustments to offer relief and restoration.

But this journey is about more than just physical well-being. It's about empowering your mindset, fostering resilience, and igniting a sense of control over your health. We'll delve into mindfulness, meditation, and the power of positivity, recognizing that true healing encompasses more than just the body.

CHAPTER ONE

UNDERSTANDING FIBROID

Fibroids, medically known as uterine leiomyomas, are benign (non-cancerous) growths that develop within the muscular walls of the uterus. While they are common, their presence and impact can vary widely among individuals. To truly understand fibroids, it's important to explore their nature, causes, symptoms, and potential effects on health. pea to as large as a grapefruit or even bigger. They can appear as a single growth or as multiple growths in the uterus. Their location within the uterus can also vary, influencing the symptoms they cause and the treatment options available

Unraveling the Causes of Fibroid

Fibroids, also known as uterine leiomyomas, are complex growths that emerge within the uterine walls. While the exact causes remain multifaceted and not fully understood, several factors are believed to contribute to their development. Here are the detailed causes that researchers have identified as potential influencers of fibroid formation.

1. Hormonal Influence: Estrogen, a female sex hormone, is thought to be a significant driver of fibroid growth. Estrogen stimulates the uterine lining during the menstrual cycle, and high levels of estrogen can encourage the proliferation of fibroid cells. Fibroids tend to grow during periods of hormonal activity, such as pregnancy, and may shrink after menopause when estrogen levels decrease.

2. Genetic Predisposition: If your immediate family members, particularly your mother or sister, have had fibroids, you may be at a higher risk of developing them. Genetic factors appear to play a role in susceptibility to fibroid growth.

3. Race and Ethnicity: Women of African descent are more likely to develop fibroids and tend to develop them at a younger age and with greater severity.

4. Lifestyle Factors: Excess body weight is associated with higher levels of estrogen, which could contribute to fibroid development. Obesity may also influence inflammation and insulin resistance, potentially affecting and fibroid growth.

5. Early Onset of Menstruation: Beginning menstruation at an early age (before 10 years old) has been associated with a higher risk of fibroids.

9. Pregnancy and Hormonal Changes: Hormonal fluctuations during pregnancy can cause the rapid

rise in estrogen therefore cause existing fibroids to grow. They usually regress after childbirth when hormone levels stabilize.

Research continues to shed light on the intricate web of influences that contribute to the growth of fibroids, allowing for more informed approaches to prevention and treatment.

Symptoms of Fibroids

Fibroids can lead to a range of symptoms, some of which may be debilitating while others are barely noticeable. Common symptoms include:

Heavy Menstrual Bleeding: Fibroids can lead to prolonged and heavy menstrual periods, causing anemia and fatigue.

Pelvic Pain and Pressure: Larger fibroids can cause discomfort and pressure in the pelvic region.

Urinary Symptoms: Fibroids pressing on the bladder can lead to frequent urination and urgency.

Bowel Symptoms: Similarly, fibroids pressing on the rectum can cause constipation and discomfort.

Abdominal Enlargement: Large fibroids can cause the uterus to expand, leading to a swollen abdomen.

Fertility and Pregnancy Impact: Depending on their location and size, fibroids can affect fertility and pregnancy outcomes.

Impact of Fibroid Symptoms on Health

The impact of fibroids on health can vary widely depending on factors such as the size, number, and location of the fibroids, as well as individual characteristics and overall health. Here's an overview of how fibroids can affect health:

1. Menstrual and Reproductive Health:

Heavy Menstrual Bleeding: One of the most common symptoms of fibroids is heavy and prolonged menstrual bleeding (menorrhagia). This can lead to anemia due to excessive blood loss, causing fatigue and weakness.

Pain and Discomfort: Fibroids can cause pelvic pain, pressure, and cramping. Severe pain may affect daily activities and quality of life.

Fertility: Depending on their location, fibroids can impact fertility. They can interfere with the implantation of a fertilized egg, affect the shape of the uterine cavity, or disrupt the normal functioning of the fallopian tubes.

Pregnancy: Fibroids can increase the risk of complications during pregnancy, including preterm labor, placental abruption, and cesarean delivery.

2. Urinary and Gastrointestinal Symptoms:

Urinary Frequency and Urgency: Large fibroids can press against the bladder, causing frequent urination and a constant feeling of urgency.

Bowel Symptoms: Fibroids located near the rectum can lead to constipation, discomfort, and a sensation of bowel fullness.

3. Physical and Emotional Well-being:

Fatigue: Chronic heavy bleeding and anemia can lead to fatigue and decreased energy levels.

Emotional Impact: Dealing with the symptoms and potential implications of fibroids, such as fertility challenges or pain, can result in stress, anxiety, and emotional distress.

Impact on Daily Activities: Severe symptoms can interfere with work, exercise, social activities, and overall quality of life.

4. Quality of Life:

Body Image: Large fibroids can cause abdominal enlargement, which may affect body image and self-esteem.

5. Sexual Function: Fibroids can lead to discomfort or pain during sexual intercourse.

It's important to note that not all fibroids cause symptoms, and some women may have fibroids without being aware of their presence. The impact of fibroids on health can range from minimal to significant. Consulting with healthcare professionals and exploring appropriate management options is crucial to addressing symptoms, maintaining reproductive health, and improving overall quality of life.

CHAPTER TWO

CLINICAL PERSPECTIVES ON FIBROID

Medical perspectives on fibroids offer insights from healthcare professionals who specialize in diagnosing, treating, and managing fibroid-related conditions. These perspectives encompass a range of approaches, from conventional treatments to emerging innovations, aiming to provide patients with effective solutions for fibroid management. Here, we delve into the key medical viewpoints surrounding fibroids

Diagnosis Process Of Fibroid

Diagnosing fibroids involves a series of steps to accurately identify the presence, size, and characteristics of these non-cancerous growths within the uterus. Healthcare professionals employ a combination of medical history, physical examinations, and advanced imaging techniques to achieve an accurate diagnosis. Here's a comprehensive breakdown of the diagnosis process:

1. Medical History:

Your healthcare provider will begin by gathering detailed information about your medical history, including any symptoms you're experiencing, menstrual patterns, previous health conditions, and family history of fibroids or reproductive issues.

2. Physical Examination:

A pelvic examination is a crucial initial step. During this examination, your healthcare provider can feel for any irregularities, changes in uterine size or shape, and the presence of masses. The examination helps determine if further diagnostic tests are necessary.

3. Imaging Techniques:

Advanced imaging techniques play a pivotal role in visualizing fibroids and providing critical information about their location, size, and characteristics. Common imaging methods include:

Ultrasound: Transabdominal or transvaginal ultrasound uses sound waves to create images of the uterus and fibroids. It's often the first imaging tool used to diagnose fibroids.

MRI (Magnetic Resonance Imaging): MRI provides detailed images that help differentiate fibroids from other uterine conditions and provides information about the number, size, and location of fibroids.

CT Scan (Computed Tomography): While less commonly used, CT scans can also offer cross-sectional images that aid in diagnosis and treatment planning.

4. Hysteroscopy:

If fibroids are suspected to be within the uterine cavity, a hysteroscope thin lighted tube is inserted through the cervix to allow direct visualization of the inside of the uterus. This procedure can help diagnose submucosal fibroids that grow into the uterine cavity.

5. Biopsy:

In some cases, if there's uncertainty about the diagnosis or if malignancy (cancer) is a concern, a biopsy might be recommended. A small tissue sample is taken from the fibroid or the uterine lining and analyzed to rule out other conditions.

6. Differential Diagnosis:

Diagnosing fibroids involves ruling out other conditions that might present with similar symptoms. Conditions like adenomyosis (thickening of the uterine lining) or ovarian cysts can mimic fibroid symptoms, so a comprehensive evaluation is crucial.

7. Consultation and Discussion:

After the diagnosis is confirmed, your healthcare provider will discuss the findings with you. They will explain the size, location, and potential impact of the fibroids on your health. Based on your symptoms, fertility goals, and overall health, you'll collaboratively decide on an appropriate treatment plan.

In summary, diagnosing fibroids involves a holistic approach that integrates medical history, physical examinations, and advanced imaging techniques.

Navigating Choices of Fibroid Treatments

The treatment of fibroids is multifaceted, considering factors such as symptom severity, reproductive goals, overall health, and personal preferences. Healthcare professionals offer a range of options, from conservative approaches to surgical interventions. Here's an overview of the diverse treatment pathways available for managing fibroids:

1. Watchful Waiting:

If fibroids are small, asymptomatic, or not significantly impacting your quality of life, your healthcare provider might recommend monitoring them without immediate intervention. Regular check-ups and imaging tests help ensure that any changes in size or symptoms are carefully tracked.

2. Medications:

Pain Relievers: Over-the-counter pain relievers, such as ibuprofen, can help manage discomfort and menstrual cramps associated with fibroids.

Hormonal Birth Control: Oral contraceptives, hormonal IUDs, and other hormonal methods can help regulate heavy menstrual bleeding and manage symptoms.

GnRH Agonists: These medications induce a temporary menopause-like state, reducing estrogen production and fibroid size. They are usually used for a short period due to side effects.

3. Minimally Invasive Procedures:

Uterine Artery Embolization (UAE): A radiologist injects tiny particles into the blood vessels that supply the fibroids, cutting off their blood flow and causing them to shrink.

Magnetic Resonance-guided Focused Ultrasound (MRgFUS): Uses focused ultrasound waves to heat and destroy fibroid tissue, while monitoring with MRI.

Laparoscopic or Robotic Myomectomy: Surgical removal of fibroids through small incisions, leaving the uterus intact.

4. Surgical Interventions:

Myomectomy: Surgical removal of fibroids while preserving the uterus. It's a good option for those who want to maintain fertility.

Hysterectomy: Complete removal of the uterus. It's a definitive solution for fibroids but is not an option for those who wish to have children.

5. Emerging Therapies:

Focused Ultrasound Ablation: Using ultrasound waves to destroy fibroids without incisions.

6.Endometrial Ablation: For smaller fibroids that mainly affect the uterine lining.

Ultimately, the treatment journey for fibroids is individualized, taking into account your unique circumstances and preferences. Open communication with your healthcare provider ensures that you receive the information and guidance needed to make informed decisions about your fibroid management plan.

Limitations and Side Effects of Conventional Fibroid Treatments

While conventional treatments for fibroids can offer relief and improved quality of life for many individuals, it's important to be aware of their limitations and potential side effects.

1. Medications:

Limitations:

Medications provide symptom relief but do not eliminate fibroids.

They may not be effective for larger fibroids or for those causing severe symptoms.

Some treatments, like GnRH agonists, are usually recommended for short-term use due to potential side effects and concerns about bone density.

Potential Side Effects:
Hormonal treatments can lead to side effects such as mood changes, hot flashes, weight gain, and breast tenderness.
GnRH agonists can induce menopause-like symptoms, including vaginal dryness, reduced libido, and bone density loss.
There may be risks associated with long-term hormonal therapies, particularly in older women.
2. Minimally Invasive Procedures:
Limitations:
The effectiveness of procedures like UAE and MRgFUS might vary based on the size, number, and location of fibroids.
Some fibroids may not be suitable for these procedures, and follow-up treatments might be necessary.
These procedures may not be recommended for women who want to preserve fertility.
Potential Side Effects:
Minimally invasive procedures can cause pain, discomfort, and a temporary increase in fibroid-related symptoms during recovery.
There's a potential risk of infection or injury to nearby organs
3. Surgical Interventions:
Limitations:

Hysterectomy is a definitive solution but is not
suitable for those who wish to maintain fertility.
Myomectomy, while preserving fertility potential,
might require more time for recovery compared to
minimally invasive procedures.
All surgeries carry risks associated with anesthesia,
bleeding, and infection.
Potential Side Effects:
Surgical procedures can lead to pain, scarring, and
a longer recovery period.
Hysterectomy results in the loss of fertility and
brings about menopause if the ovaries are
removed.

CHAPTER THREE

LIFESTYLE MODIFICATION TOWARDS NURTURING WELLNESS

A holistic approach to fibroid healing acknowledges that physical health is deeply interconnected with emotional, mental, and spiritual well-being. This comprehensive strategy encompasses various elements that promote overall health while addressing the specific challenges posed by fibroids. Here's an exploration of the key components of the holistic approach to fibroid healing:

1. Nutrition and Diet:

Emphasis on a balanced and nutrient-rich diet that supports hormonal balance and overall well-being. Consume whole foods, such as fruits, vegetables, whole grains, lean proteins, and healthy fats. Reduction of processed foods, excess sugar, caffeine, and alcohol, which can disrupt hormone equilibrium.

Phytoestrogen-Rich Foods: Incorporate foods rich in phytoestrogen like cruciferous vegetables, flaxseeds, and legumes to support hormonal balance.

Anti-Inflammatory Foods: Choose foods rich in antioxidants and omega-3 fatty acids to reduce inflammation.

2. Stress Management and Mindfulness:

Utilization of stress reduction techniques, such as meditation, deep breathing, and mindfulness to manage stress hormones. Engage in activities that bring you joy and emotional fulfillment.

3. Physical Activity:

Regular exercise like walking, jogging, swimming and cycling enhances weight management, and reduce inflammation. Exercises that specifically target the pelvic area can improve blood flow and alleviate discomfort

Engage in activities that bring you joy and emotional fulfillment.

Yoga and Pilates are practices combine physical movement, deep breathing, and relaxation techniques, promoting stress reduction and flexibility.

4. Herbal Remedies and Supplements:

Utilization of specific herbs and supplements that are believed to support hormone balance and fibroid management. Consult with your healthcare provider before introducing new supplements or herbs into the routine.

5. Sleep Quality:

Prioritization of quality sleep to facilitate hormonal regulation and overall recovery.

Creating a bedtime routine and optimizing a sleep environment to ensure adequate sleep.

6. Emotional and Psychological Support:

Recognition of the emotional impact of fibroids and seeking support from friends, family, or therapists. Engaging in activities that bring joy, creativity, and emotional fulfillment.

7. Education and Empowerment:

Reduction of exposure to environmental toxins that may disrupt balance hormone.

Empowering individuals to take an active role in their healing journey.

Understanding that every individual's healing journey is unique.

By embracing a comprehensive strategy that addresses all these dimensions, individuals can navigate their fibroid journey with a sense of empowerment, resilience, and improved overall well-being.

Stress, Hormones, and Fibroid Growth

The intricate relationship between the mind and body extends to the growth of fibroids, as stress and hormonal influences interplay to impact their development and progression. This mind-body connection sheds light on how stress, hormones, and

fibroid growth are interconnected, influencing each other in a complex dance. Here's an in-depth exploration of their fascinating relationship:

1. Stress Hormones and Fibroid Growth:
Stress Response: When the body perceives stress, it triggers the release of stress hormones, primarily cortisol and adrenaline. This "fight or flight" response prepares the body for immediate action in the face of danger.

Impact on hormones: Chronic stress can disrupt the delicate balance of hormones in the body. Stress hormones, particularly cortisol, can interfere with the regular production of reproductive hormones, such as estrogen and progesterone. This disruption can lead to hormonal imbalances that may contribute to fibroid growth.

2. Estrogen Dominance and Fibroid Development:
Estrogen's Role: Estrogen, a primary female sex hormone, plays a significant role in the development of fibroids. It stimulates the growth of the uterine lining during the menstrual cycle and promotes cell proliferation.

Chronic stress can lead to a phenomenon known as "estrogen dominance," where there is an excess of estrogen relative to progesterone. This hormonal imbalance is linked to increased fibroid growth, as estrogen encourages the proliferation of fibroid cells.

3. Inflammation and Fibroid Growth:
Inflammatory Response: Stress triggers an inflammatory response in the body. While inflammation is a natural defense mechanism, chronic inflammation can contribute to the development and growth of fibroids.
Influence on Blood Flow: Inflammation can lead to blood vessel constriction and reduced blood flow to certain areas, including the uterus. Diminished blood flow may impact the oxygen and nutrient supply to uterine tissues, potentially fostering fibroid growth.

4. Cortisol's Role:
Impact of cortisol: Excessive cortisol production, characteristic of chronic stress, can negatively affect the body's ability to regulate inflammation and manage tissue repair.
Cell Proliferation: Cortisol can stimulate cell proliferation, which may be a contributing factor in fibroid development. Elevated cortisol levels could enhance the growth of fibroid tissue.
5. Feedback Loop:
Cyclic Nature: Stress, hormones, and fibroid growth form a cyclic relationship. Stress can disrupt hormonal balance, leading to estrogen dominance and potentially fueling fibroid growth. In turn, the

presence of fibroids can cause discomfort and emotional distress, creating additional stress.

Understanding this intricate interplay underscores the importance of stress management in fibroid prevention and management. By nurturing the mind-body connection, individuals can potentially influence their hormonal equilibrium and contribute to their overall well-being, thus shaping their fibroid journey in a more positive direction.

Role of Nutrition in Managing Fibroids

Nutrition plays a crucial role in managing fibroids, as the foods we consume can influence hormonal balance, inflammation, and overall well-being. By making mindful dietary choices, individuals can potentially support their bodies in maintaining hormonal equilibrium and reducing the impact of fibroids. Here's a closer look at the role of nutrition in managing fibroids:

1. Hormonal Balance:
Phytoestrogen: Certain plant compounds called phytoestrogen have a mild estrogen-like effect in the body. Including foods rich in phytoestrogen, such as soy, flaxseeds, and legumes, can help modulate estrogen levels, potentially reducing the

impact of estrogen dominance that may contribute to fibroid growth.

Balanced Macronutrients: A balanced diet that includes adequate protein, healthy fats, and complex carbohydrates supports stable blood sugar levels. Balanced blood sugar can help prevent insulin spikes, which can affect hormone regulation.

2. Anti-Inflammatory Effects:

Omega-3 Fatty Acids: Foods rich in omega-3 fatty acids, like fatty fish (salmon, mackerel, sardines), walnuts, and chia seeds, have anti-inflammatory properties. Chronic inflammation is believed to contribute to fibroid growth, so consuming anti-inflammatory foods may have a positive impact.

Antioxidant-Rich Foods: Brightly colored fruits and vegetables, such as berries, leafy greens, and citrus fruits, are high in antioxidants. Antioxidants help combat oxidative stress and inflammation, potentially supporting fibroid management.

3. Iron Intake and Anemia:

Iron-Rich Foods: Fibroids can cause heavy menstrual bleeding, leading to an increased risk of iron deficiency anemia. Consuming iron-rich foods, such as lean meats, dark leafy greens, lentils, and fortified cereals, can help prevent anemia.

4. Fiber for Hormone Metabolism:

Dietary Fiber: A diet high in fiber supports healthy digestion and promotes the excretion of excess hormones. Whole grains, legumes, fruits, and vegetables are excellent sources of dietary fiber.

Herbal Remedies and Supplements for Nurturing wellness

Herbal remedies and supplements are often considered as complementary options for managing fibroids, aiming to support hormonal balance, reduce symptoms, and promote healing. It's important to note that while some individuals may find relief from these natural approaches, their efficacy can vary. Before incorporating any herbal remedies or supplements, consult with a healthcare provider, especially if you have underlying health conditions or taking medications. Here's an in-depth look at some commonly used herbal remedies and supplements for fibroid management:

1. Vitex (Chaste Tree Berry): Vitex is believed to influence hormonal balance by affecting the pituitary gland and regulating the production of various hormones, including prolactin and progesterone. It may help reduce heavy bleeding and alleviate symptoms related to hormonal imbalances.

2. Milk Thistle: Milk thistle is known for its liver-supporting properties. It aids the liver in processing hormones and toxins from the body. Improved liver

function may aid in hormone metabolism, potentially benefiting individuals with estrogen dominance.

3. DIM (Diindolylmethane): DIM is derived from cruciferous vegetables. It supports estrogen metabolism by promoting the breakdown of estrogen into less potent forms. By assisting in estrogen metabolism, DIM may help balance hormone levels and reduce the impact of estrogen dominance.

4. Turmeric: Turmeric contains curcumin, a compound with anti-inflammatory and antioxidant properties. Curcumin's anti-inflammatory effects may help mitigate the inflammation associated with fibroid growth.

5. Evening Primrose Oil: Evening primrose oil contains gamma-linolenic acid (GLA), an essential fatty acid that plays a role in hormone regulation. Potential Benefits: GLA may help regulate hormonal balance and manage symptoms like breast tenderness and mood fluctuations.

6. Green Tea Extract: Green tea is rich in antioxidants, particularly epigallocatechin gallate (EGCG). EGCG's antioxidant properties may help reduce oxidative stress and inflammation associated with fibroid growth.

7. Black Cohosh: Black cohosh is traditionally used for hormonal balance, particularly in menopausal

women. It may help alleviate symptoms related to hormonal fluctuations, such as heavy bleeding and mood changes.

8. Omega-3 Fatty Acids: Omega-3 fatty acids have anti-inflammatory properties. Reducing inflammation may contribute to managing symptoms related to fibroids.

9. Iron Supplements: Iron supplements help prevent or address anemia resulting from heavy menstrual bleeding. Maintaining adequate iron level supports overall energy and well-being.

10. Herbal Teas: Certain herbal teas, such as raspberry leaf, nettle, and ginger tea, are believed to support uterine health and hormone balance. These teas may provide comfort and potential benefits, although scientific evidence is limited.

Remember that individual responses to herbal remedies and supplements can vary. It's crucial to consult a healthcare provider before incorporating these options into your routine. Herbal remedies and supplements should not replace conventional medical treatments, especially in cases where symptoms are severe or fibroid growth is significant.

Complementary Practices To Enhance Wellness

Complementary practices such as acupuncture, and other holistic approaches play a vital role in managing fibroids by promoting relaxation, reducing stress, and enhancing overall well-being. These practices offer a holistic perspective that addresses the mind, body, and spirit. Below are complementary practices that contribute to fibroid management:

1. Acupuncture:
Role: Acupuncture involves inserting thin needles into specific points on the body to stimulate energy flow.
Potential Benefits: Acupuncture is believed to promote blood circulation, reduce inflammation, and stimulate the body's natural healing processes. It may help alleviate pain, discomfort, and stress associated with fibroids.

2. Yoga:
Role: Yoga combines physical postures, breathing exercises, and meditation to promote physical and mental well-being.
Potential Benefits: Yoga supports flexibility, reduces stress, improves circulation, and enhances mind-body awareness. Specific yoga poses can target

the pelvic region, promoting blood flow and relaxation.

3. Meditation:
Role: Meditation and mindfulness practices cultivate present-moment awareness and promote relaxation.
Potential Benefits: These practices reduce stress, anxiety, and emotional distress, potentially influencing hormonal balance and reducing inflammation.

4. Tai Chi and Qigong:
Role: Tai Chi and Qigong involve slow, flowing movements and deep breathing exercises.
Potential Benefits: These practices promote relaxation, balance, and energy flow. They can support stress reduction and overall well-being.

5.Aromatherapy:
Role: Aromatherapy involves using essential oils to promote relaxation and well-being.
Potential Benefits: Certain essential oils, such as lavender and chamomile, can support stress reduction and emotional balance.

6.Massage Therapy:

Role: Massage therapy promotes relaxation, improves blood circulation, and reduces muscle tension.
Potential Benefits: Regular massages can contribute to stress reduction and alleviate physical discomfort.

7. Guided Imagery:
Role: Guided imagery involves visualizing positive scenarios to promote relaxation and manage stress.
Potential Benefits: This practice enhances relaxation, reduces stress, and can positively influence emotional well-being.

8 Consultation with Professionals:
Guidance: Seek guidance from qualified practitioners, such as licensed acupuncturists, certified yoga instructors, and healthcare providers.

While these complementary practices can offer numerous benefits for fibroid management, it's important to remember that individual responses may vary. Always consult with healthcare professionals before incorporating new practices, especially if you have existing health conditions or are taking medications. Integrating these approaches as part of a holistic strategy can enhance your fibroid management journey and contribute to your overall well-being.

CHAPTER FOUR

EMPOWERING YOUR MINDSET

Empowering your mindset involves adopting positive change and proactive approach to life's challenges, including those posed by fibroids. By nurturing a resilient and optimistic mindset, you can enhance your ability to navigate the journey of fibroid management and improve your overall well-being. Here's how to cultivate an empowered mindset:

1.Acknowledge your emotions and thoughts without judgment.Accepting your feelings allows you to process them and move forward.
2. Focus on What You Can Control, direct your energy towards aspects you can influence, such as your lifestyle, mindset, and reactions to challenges.
3. Replace self-criticism with self-compassion and positive affirmations. Treat yourself with the same kindness you'd offer a friend.
4. Embrace setbacks as opportunities for growth. Cultivate resilience by learning from challenges and adapting to new situations.
5. Practice living in the moment tin order to reducing anxiety about the future.
6. Setting Goals and Celebrating Progress:
Set achievable goals related to your healing journey and celebrate every step forward.
7 Education and Empowerment, learn about fibroids and available treatments to make informed decisions about your health.

8. Cultivate gratitude for the positive aspects of your life. Focus on what you have rather than what you lack.

9. Visualize your desired outcomes and engage in relaxation techniques to alleviate stress.

10. Prioritize self-care activities that bring you joy, relaxation, and rejuvenation.

11. Be patient with yourself as you navigate challenges. Show yourself the same compassion you'd extend to others.

12. Seek Professional Guidance If needed, work with therapists or counselors who specialize in stress management and mindset development.

13. Recognize that change and adaptation is part of life. Embrace a flexible mindset that allows you to adapt to new situations and challenges.

14. Develop a Support System. Surround yourself with friends, family, or support groups that offer understanding, empathy, and a sense of community.

15. Remember that transforming your mindset is a gradual process. Empowering your health not only contributes to better fibroid management, but also enriches your quality of life.

Building resilience and fostering positive mental health is a lifelong journey. By incorporating these strategies into your daily life, you'll enhance your ability to navigate fibroid-related challenges and embrace the broader journey of well-being. Remember that seeking professional support when needed is a sign of strength and a valuable step towards nurturing your mental health.

Exploring Energy Healing and Its Potential Benefits

Energy healing is a whole practice that focuses on channeling and balancing the body's energy to promote physical, emotional, and spiritual well-being. While scientific research on energy healing is still evolving, many individuals have reported positive experiences and benefits. Here's an overview of energy healing and its potential benefits:

1. Types of Energy Healing:
Reiki: Involves a practitioner using their hands to transfer healing energy to the recipient, promoting relaxation and balance.
Chakra Healing: Focuses on the body's energy centers (chakras) to remove blockages and restore energy flow.
Pranic Healing: Involves manipulating the body's energy (prana) to promote healing and well-being.
Healing Touch: Utilizes gentle touch to clear energy blockages and promote relaxation.

2. Potential Benefits of Energy Healing:
Stress Reduction: Energy healing techniques often induce a state of deep relaxation, reducing stress and promoting emotional well-being.
Pain Relief: Some individuals have reported pain reduction and increased comfort after energy healing sessions.
Emotional Balance: Energy healing may help alleviate emotional distress, anxiety, and depression by promoting a sense of calm.
Enhanced Vitality: Practitioners often report increased energy levels and a sense of vitality after energy healing sessions.
Immune System Support: Improved energy flow is believed to support the body's natural healing mechanisms.
Holistic Approach: Energy healing considers the mind, body, and spirit as interconnected, promoting a comprehensive sense of well-being.

3. Mind-Body Connection:
Energy healing practices are rooted in the idea that imbalances in the body's energy can manifest as physical or emotional ailments.
By rebalancing the body's energy, energy healing aims to address underlying causes rather than just managing symptoms.

4. Individual Experience:

Responses to energy healing can vary widely. Some individuals experience immediate relief, while others may notice gradual improvements over time.

5. Complementary Practice:
Energy healing can be used alongside conventional medical treatments as a complementary approach, rather than a replacement.
Consulting with healthcare providers before incorporating energy healing is advisable, especially if you have existing health conditions or are undergoing medical treatments.

6. Ethical Considerations:
Ensure that your chosen practitioner adheres to ethical standards and practices.

7. Placebo Effect:
It's worth noting that some reported benefits of energy healing might be attributed to the placebo effect, where the belief in a treatment's effectiveness influences the outcome.

8. Personal Exploration:
If you're curious about energy healing, consider exploring it with an open mind. Be prepared for a diverse range of experiences and outcomes.

While energy healing may not be a universally accepted practice within the medical community, many individuals find value in its potential benefits. As with any holistic approach, it's important to approach energy healing with an informed and discerning perspective, seeking guidance from qualified practitioners and healthcare professionals when needed.

Healing Words of Affirmation

Certainly, here are some healing words of affirmation to inspire and uplift you on your journey:

1.I am strong, resilient, and capable of healing.

2.I release any negative energy and embrace the healing power within me.

3.Every day, I am taking steps towards my well-being and vitality.

4.My body is a vessel of healing and transformation.

5.I trust in the wisdom of my body to guide me towards optimal health.

6.I love, care, and healing.

7.I am in tune with my body's needs, and I honor them with compassion.

8.I embrace each challenge as an opportunity for growth and healing.

9.I am the author of my health journey, and I write a story of wellness and empowerment.

10. I am surrounded by love, support, and positive energy on my path to healing.

11. I release fear and welcome peace and healing into my life.

12. I am grateful for every step of progress on my healing journey.

13. I radiate positivity, and my body responds with vibrant health.

14. I am connected to the healing energy of the universe, and it flows through me.

15. My body knows how to heal, and I trust in its innate wisdom.

16. I am open to receiving the abundance of health and well-being that is available to me.

17. I am not defined by my challenges; I am defined by my strength and resilience.

18. With each breath, I inhale healing energy and exhale any discomfort.

19. I am a source of light and healing for myself and those around me.

20. I embrace the journey of healing with patience, grace, and determination.

Repeat these affirmations regularly, allow their positive energy to uplift your spirit and support your healing journey. Remember, your mindset plays a powerful role in your well-being, and these affirmations can help you foster a positive and healing outlook.

CHAPTER FIVE

LOOKING AHEAD: THE FUTURE OF FIBROID TREATMENT

Advancements in medical research and technology would continue to shape the future of fibroid treatment, offering new possibilities for more effective and patient-centered approaches. Here are some trends and potential directions that could shape the future of fibroid treatment:

1. Minimally Invasive Techniques
The trend toward minimally invasive surgical techniques,
such as laparoscopic and robotic-assisted surgeries, is
likely to continue. These methods offer quicker recovery
times and less scarring compared to traditional open
surgeries.

2. Targeted Therapies
Developing treatments that specifically target fibroid
cells while minimizing impact on healthy tissue remains
a focus. Targeted therapies could potentially reduce
side effects and improve outcomes.

3. Non-Invasive Options
Non-invasive procedures like focused ultrasound
(MRgFUS) and radio-frequency ablation are becoming
more refined. These approaches can provide
alternatives to surgery while minimizing risks and
recovery time.

4. Personalized Medicine
Advances in genetics and personalized medicine could
lead to treatments tailored to an individual's unique
genetic and hormonal makeup, potentially improving
treatment outcomes and reducing side effects.

5. Hormonal Therapies
Ongoing research into hormonal therapies aims to
develop treatments that effectively manage fibroid
growth while minimizing hormonal imbalances and
associated symptoms.

6. Alternative Therapies
The integration of complementary and alternative
therapies, such as acupuncture, yoga, and herbal
remedies, could become more mainstream as their
benefits are further explored.

7. Fertility Preservation
As more women delay childbearing, there's a growing
interest in fibroid treatments that prioritize fertility
preservation, ensuring that women have options to
conceive and carry pregnancies.

8. Patient-Centered Care
The future of fibroid treatment may involve more patient-
centered and shared decision-making approaches.
Patients will have a more active role in their treatment
plans and options.

9. Remote Monitoring and Telemedicine
Remote monitoring technologies and telemedicine
platforms may become more prevalent, allowing patients
to track their fibroid status and consult with healthcare
providers without frequent in-person visits.

10. Research and Clinical Trials
Continued research and clinical trials will drive
innovation in fibroid treatment, potentially uncovering
new approaches that offer improved outcomes and
quality of life.

It's important to note that the future of fibroid treatment will likely be influenced by ongoing research, regulatory approvals, and evolving medical practices. As you navigate your fibroid journey, staying informed about the latest advancements and discussing potential treatment options with your healthcare provider will empower you to make well-informed decisions about your care.

Innovations, Research, and Emerging Solutions in Fibroid Management

Advancements in medical research and technology are continuously shaping the landscape of fibroid management. Emerging solutions and innovations offer promising alternatives and improvements in treatment options. Here are some innovations, research areas, and potential emerging solutions in fibroid management:

1. Radio frequency Ablation and Focused Ultrasound:
These non-invasive techniques use heat or ultrasound waves to destroy fibroid tissue while preserving surrounding healthy tissue. They offer a less invasive option for fibroid removal.

2. Uterine Artery Embolization (UAE):
UAE involves blocking the blood supply to fibroids, causing them to shrink. Ongoing research aims to optimize this technique for various fibroid types.

3. Hormonal Therapies:
Research is focusing on hormonal therapies that manage fibroid growth without significant hormonal side effects, providing a more balanced approach to treatment.

4. Genetic and Molecular Research:
Understanding the genetic and molecular basis of
fibroids could lead to targeted therapies that directly
address the factors contributing to their growth.
5. Medication Advancements:
Ongoing research explores new medication options that
specifically target fibroid growth factors, reducing the
need for surgery.
6. Personalized Treatment Plans:
The integration of patient data, genetics, and medical
history could lead to personalized treatment plans
tailored to each individual's needs.
7. Telemedicine and Remote Monitoring:
Telemedicine platforms and remote monitoring tools
allow patients to receive care and consultation without
frequent in-person visits.
8. Patient-Centered Care:
Healthcare providers are increasingly focusing on
patient preferences, quality of life, and shared decision-
making in treatment plans.
9.Advancements in Anesthesia:
Improved anesthesia techniques ensure patient comfort
during minimally invasive procedures.
10. Regenerative Medicine:
Research into regenerative medicine may lead to the
development of therapies that promote the natural
healing and restoration of uterine tissue.
As research progresses, these innovations hold the
potential to transform the field of fibroid management,
offering more options, improved outcomes, and
enhanced quality of life for individuals with fibroids.

Staying informed about these advancements and discussing potential treatment options with your healthcare provider will empower you to make informed decisions about your fibroid management journey.

CONCLUSION

In the journey towards "Fibroid Freedom: Empowering Women's wellness through Natural approach and Holistic Healing." We've delved deep into the realm of fibroids, exploring their causes, impact, and the array of strategies to manage them effectively. From medical perspectives and diagnosis to conventional and holistic treatments, we've uncovered a wealth of knowledge to guide you towards informed decisions.

Fibroids need not be an obstacle,they can be a catalyst for personal growth and empowerment. As you stand at the crossroads of your fibroid journey, armed with knowledge, resilience, and a proactive approach, you're ready to embark on a path towards Fibroid Freedom. Remember, empowerment comes not only from the strategies you've learned, but from the newfound confidence to advocate for your health, make informed decisions, and shape a future of vitality and well-being. The journey continues, and as you step forward, may "Fibroid Freedom" serve as a guiding light, empowering you to take charge of your health and embrace a life of empowerment and well-being.

www.ingramcontent.com/pod-product-compliance
Lightning Source LLC
Chambersburg PA
CBHW070735260726

48660CB00007B/2862